Binge Eating

Binge Eating Guide to Stop and Overcome Overeating

Table of Contents

Introduction

Chapter 1: Identifying and Overcoming the Causes Of Bingeing

Chapter 2: Managing Your Food

Chapter 3: Put an End To Dieting and Other Bad Habits

Chapter 4: Create Sustainable Eating and Living Habits

Chapter 5: Self Acceptance and Avoiding Relapse

Conclusion

© Copyright 2018 by Charlie Mason - All rights reserved.

The following Book is reproduced below with the goal of providing information that is as accurate and reliable as possible. Regardless, purchasing this Book can be seen as consent to the fact that both the publisher and the author of this book are in no way experts on the topics discussed within and that any recommendations or suggestions that are made herein are for entertainment purposes only. Professionals should be consulted as needed prior to undertaking any of the action endorsed herein.

This declaration is deemed fair and valid by both the American Bar Association and the Committee of Publishers Association and is legally binding throughout the United States.

Furthermore, the transmission, duplication or reproduction of any of the following work including specific information will be considered an illegal act irrespective of if it is done electronically or in print. This extends to creating a secondary or tertiary copy of the work or a recorded copy and is only allowed with express written consent from the Publisher. All additional rights reserved.

The information in the following pages is broadly considered to be a truthful and accurate account of facts and as such any inattention, use or misuse of the information in question by the reader will render any resulting actions solely under their purview. There are no scenarios in which the publisher or the original author of this work can be in any fashion deemed liable for any hardship or damages that may befall them after undertaking information described herein.

Additionally, the information in the following pages is intended only for informational purposes and should thus be thought of as universal. As befitting its nature, it is presented without assurance regarding its prolonged validity or interim quality. Trademarks that are mentioned are done without written consent and can in no way be considered an endorsement from the trademark holder.

Introduction

Congratulations on purchasing the *Binge Eating: Guide to Stop and Overcome Overeating* and thank you for doing so. Obesity is omnipresent today. In many cities over half of the adults are obese, and many of the children are as well. One of the largest contributors to obesity is binge eating. Binge eating is when someone is driven to eat compulsively and keeps eating passed the point of fullness and even passed the point of physical pain. It is often done in an altered state of consciousness in which the eater doesn't even notice what she/he is eating. Binge eating, quite often, is a contributing factor to the diabetes epidemic.

The following chapters will discuss the causes of binge eating and learn how to stop it. By learning what triggers a binge eating episode, a person is empowered to break the cycle that keeps them unhealthy and unhappy. Also explained is why diets will not make you thinner nor stop overeating. The bad habits that keep you locked into continuing binge eating are described along with an easy way to do away with them. A guide to making a food plan that will give you complete control over your food intake is included. Finally, a chapter devoted to strategies for continued success in avoiding binge eating and its associated maladies.

There are plenty of books on this subject on the market, thanks again for choosing this one! Every effort was made to ensure it is full of as much useful information as possible, please enjoy!

As a way of saying thank you for purchasing my book, please use your link below to claim your 3 FREE Cookbooks on Health, Fitness & Dieting Instantly

https://bit.ly/2Lvj2Pm

You can also share your link with your friends and families whom you think that can benefit from the cookbooks or you can forward them the link as a gift!

Chapter 1: **Identifying and Overcoming Causes of Bingeing**

You tell yourself you aren't going to give in this time. You just need to be a little bit stronger. It's just a question of will power. You hold out for a while, and then give in to the urge to binge. Cookies, ice cream, fried rice, tacos- it doesn't matter. Even though it is food that you love, you don't particularly enjoy it. You mindlessly eat it. Maybe all at once or maybe you pick at it all day. You might not even remember eating it afterward. Finally, you start to feel sick and over full. But you keep eating. Just a little more... and then you can't eat anymore. There is physically no room left in your stomach. Unable to eat anymore, all that is left is to get rid of the evidence and begin the self loathing and shame cycle. This is what it is like to be binge eating.

Bingeing is compulsive behavior. It is ritualized and patterned. It is driven by the subconscious. You have little control over it. The urge to binge can be all consuming. It doesn't begin and end with over eating. It is a cycle, a system that perpetuates itself. There is a trigger, an eating session, and then shame and feeling sick. These after effects leave you more susceptible to starting the cycle over again and again.

There are serious repercussions to binge eating. Obesity and diabetes are most often associated with bingeing. Each comes with potentially overwhelming health and monetary costs. There are long term mental health complications that arise from binge eating also. Negative body image and shame associated with eating disorders can spur depression and feelings of helplessness. Aside from the serious long term effects, there are immediate effects too. Nausea, abdominal pain, and low energy have an impact on quality of life, as does the ill feeling that comes from putting your body through a binge.

The cause of binge eating is not known. It is likely a combination of psychological, environmental, and biological factors- all acting on the subconscious mind. The act of bingeing is done in an altered state of consciousness. Because these are both areas largely out of our conscious control, the best way to fix the problem is to deal with something we have some control over: triggers.

Anything can serve as a trigger. There are probably as many triggers as there are people. It just depends on the individual what will or will not spur them to binge. It could be smell, a thought, stress at work or home, or even just a bad habit.

Recognizing your triggers is necessary to interrupt the cycle and stop binge eating.

Some triggers are easily recognizable. The most obvious is hunger. It is the most obvious, and the hardest to overcome in the moment. The hungrier you are the more food you will make/order, and the more you will eat. In fact, being hungry all but guarantees that you turn your next meal into a session of overeating followed by feeling ill and being ashamed.

Not all triggers are obvious. Many are hidden within our psyches and even into our metabolic function. Meaning your body is triggering itself to overeat and binge. Dehydration can be a trigger. Sometimes the body sends a message to consume water by making you thirsty. But because all food contains some water, the body can also signal you to eat to replenish water stores.

Low levels of necessary nutrients in the system my lead to binge eating, as the body calls for more food replace them. Whatever the trigger, knowing about them is the first step in dealing with them.

Not getting enough sleep can make you less alert and therefore more susceptible to over eating. When you don't feel well you can make poor decisions and get caught in a bingeing cycle. By itself, lack of sleep can cause weight gain. Add in binge eating and you can see how sleep deprivation rally works against you in your pursuit of better health.

Many triggers may be hard to avoid, like stress. You never know when you will have trouble at work or with a spouse. The world is a stressful place and random undesirable things happen. How do you avoid the unavoidable? You don't. There are a variety of stress reducing things you can do to calm yourself. Meditation, exercise, breathing exercises, or some other method may be used to keep you from overeating.

Mental health can also trigger over eating. Depression and other mental health issues can cause us to binge eat. Food can be used to self medicate. It soothes and elates us the same way that drugs do. It makes sense that we would try to alleviate the anguish of mental illness with food leading to the need for help from mental health care professionals.

The single best way to end the urge to binge is to recognize the triggers and traps that lead us into bingeing and other undesirable behavior. Knowing what your triggers are gives you the first bit of control over binge eating. Putting that knowledge to work is the next step in the battle. Practice walking away from triggers that apply to you. Make not getting caught in these traps a habit. The more you do it the easier it becomes. Keeping yourself fed and hydrated. Choosing higher quality fresh foods whenever possible to maximize health and well being is the key to sustaining a binge free life. Take care of yourself and make an effort to stay fit and active. Be sure to get enough sleep. Sleep deprivation can spur weight gain and declining health, which put you at increased risk from triggers. With enough self care, unhealthy eating habits and their effects can be minimized.

Chapter 2: Manage your food

We eat food in order to make energy for ourselves to do all the things necessary to survival and to replenish the raw materials needed to build and repair the tissues of the body. Unfortunately, many of the foods we eat today are very high in calories, and very low in nutrients. This has led to a population that is both obese and malnourished! In addition to obesity, the food we eat is causing diabetes, and general poor health. For the binge eater, the effects of this diet are multiplied.

The foods consumed during binge eating tend to be almost exclusively the worst parts of an already unhealthy diet. Bingeing on the extremely high calorie foods like processed sweets, fatty meats, and fried foods can add a full days worth of calories in only a few minutes. Eating these sugary processed foods can be catastrophic to a person's health. It gets worse. There are at least three ways in which processed foods can *cause* or, at least facilitate, binge eating.

Blood Sugar Spike

Foods that are high in refined sugar as well as simple carbohydrates (bleached flour products) are very easily metabolized by the digestive system. They can be broken down into glucose (blood sugar) in just a few minutes. Glucose is the fuel we use to power our bodies systems. The levels of glucose in our blood spikes when we eat sugars and simple carbohydrates because the body breaks them down into fuel which is deposited into the bloodstream very quickly. In other words, we get a big shot of fuel available to us... too much, in fact, to use all at once. The body reacts to high blood sugar by releasing insulin, which starts the process of storing that excess energy as fat. As the glucose levels go down, so does our energy. This cycle of extremely high blood sugar followed by extremely low blood sugar is what causes diabetes. It can also trigger and eating binge. When our blood sugar gets really low, eating again brings it back up. The body sends signals that compel us to eat, and overeating is often the result. This is a feedback loop of cause and effect that is very easy to get caught in, and can be difficult to get out of.

Quality foods like fresh fruits and vegetables, lean meats, and fish, are harder for the body to break down and extract energy from. The result is slower rise in blood sugar without the unhealthy spike. The sugars extracted from good food slowly trickle into the blood stream and provide consistent energy for hours, rather than minutes. Think of it as the difference between throwing a log on a fire and throwing a can of gas on a fire. The gas will release huge amounts of energy, but it will all be gone in a few seconds. The log will continue to burn and provide heat for a long time.

Processed Foods are Nutrient Poor

Another aspect of the fast food/boxed food diet is that is generally low in nutrients necessary to good health. Processing foods, such as milling, boiling, and preserving, strips away valuable vitamins, minerals, and other nutrients. Our bodies react to the lack of nutrients by insisting we eat more in order to recoup them. Another self perpetuating cycle- the foods we eat don't nourish us and our bodies demand more of them, even when we are not hungry, in a vain attempt to replenish nutrient stores. Many processed foods contain chemical additives which are not digestible. In order to get rid of these chemicals, the body depletes itself further of necessary nutrients to eliminate the additives.

Nutrient rich foods replace the stores of vitamins and minerals the body needs. This is why eating a healthy quality meal satisfies without necessarily feeling full. The body was lacking in nutrients, not calories.

Sugar is Addictive

Probably the most insidious aspect to a diet high in sugar is that it can be highly addictive. More and more, scientists are coming around to the evidence that sugar can be as addictive as hard drugs such as cocaine. Sugar, in high doses, alters brain chemistry the same way that cocaine and heroin do. Like other addictive drugs, the more sugar is ingested, the more you want to eat. It is yet another cyclical pattern that reinforces itself in the binge eater.

Limiting or avoiding processed sugar is the best way to deal with the addiction. But more important that removing foods from your diet is adding in as much nutrient dense food as your body needs to grow, heal, and power itself. Foods like lean meats, fresh fruits and vegetables, fish, nuts, and seeds will give you all the building blocks and consistent energy you need. It's not a question of choosing good food over bad food. If you eat good foods that you like and that are healthy, you will likely find that you want less of the processed food.

Deciding when to eat can be as important as what to eat. Meals should be spaced out to minimize hunger. Hunger is the worst trigger of all for binge eating. If you are ravenously hungry, there is very little possibility of avoiding an eating binge. An ideal schedule would have breakfast served as late in the morning as possible- but not so late that hunger pangs cause you to over eat. The later that breakfast is eaten, the longer the "fasting period" between dinner the night before and breakfast. The longer the fasting period is, the more calories are consumed. Similarly, eating dinner earlier will lengthen the fasting period thereby promoting weight loss. Again, dinner shouldn't be so early that you get hungry again before bed, because that will eventually lead to overeating.

Controlling what foods you eat and when you eat them can alleviate many of the factors that lead to binge eating. Switching to a high quality food diet that limits the intake of processed foods will do the most to help you live a healthier life.

Chapter 3: **Put an End to Dieting and Other Bad Habits**

Fad diets don't work. Most diets will help you lose weight in the short term. But the overwhelming majority of people gain all the lost weight back. Often they gain back more than they lost in the first place. Diets are usual very restrictive in both the types of foods you can eat and in quantity. It can be hard work to stay on a diet. Especially if you don't enjoy the types of foods you are allowed to eat. Diets feel like punishment, and eventually we walk away from them and into the waiting arms of a food binge.

Diets are designed to fail. We think of diets as temporary suffering that we can stop once we lose the weight we want to be rid of. So even if you do manage to lose every ounce of weight you wanted to lose, there is nothing to keep you from gaining it all back once you stop the diet. Few people make it even that far. Diets are usually broken long before weight loss goals are met. Failing at a diet makes us feel weak and hopeless. Dieting is a one of many bad habits that lead to binge eating.

Food addictions, like drug and alcohol addiction, can be very difficult to control. Habits, on the other hand are relatively easy to change. Habits form out of repetition and routine. There is little if any emotional attachment to a habit. Undoing a bad habit can be as simple as doing something else over and over until it becomes habitual. A few common bad habits that feed over eating are:

Waiting Too Long to Eat

You think that if you hold out and wait before eating you will lose more weight. Or maybe you just lost track of time and didn't realize it until you were very hungry. Either way you are now likely to overeat. It is next to impossible to not to when you are a binge eater. This habit is easily broken by planning meal times and having food prepared and ready to go.

Free Day (binge day)

Some people believe that allowing yourself to binge periodically will get the urge out of your system. One day a week you allow yourself to eat whatever you want in whatever quantities. This is a bad idea because it reinforces the idea that binge eating is an acceptable sometimes. Very quickly it will start happening more often and then everyday is potentially a free day.

Eating in the Car

We all do it, but it is a bad habit, especially for binge eaters. In the car you are insulated from the outside world and you can eat in private. This is exactly how many people prefer to binge eat. The types of foods you eat in the car are almost entirely processed packaged or fast food. So even if you don't binge in the car, the foods you eat there are sure to be empty calories at best.

Nothing but Processed Food in the House

Eating only processed foods can cause overeating as discussed in the previous chapter. Having only these types of foods on hand means that is what you will eat when you get hungry. You should always have good foods readily available.

Eating Foods We Do Not Like

We think that in order to lose weight and get healthy, we have to suffer. Part of that suffering is eating foods we don't like because they are good for us. If you get hungry and only have kale in the house to eat, you may well end up going out and getting fast food. Buy and eat healthy foods that you want to eat.

Thinking of Exercise as Punishment

We tend to think of exercise as penance for over eating. When we think of it this way, it is drudgery. You have to force yourself to go, and you can't wait for it to be over. It doesn't take long before you stop going entirely. Exercise, like healthy foods, must be enjoyable for there to be any chance of you sticking with them. Choose something you enjoy doing for exercise. Being active is one of the best things you can do for yourself. Find something you like and do it.

Snacking

Snacking can be an effective way to curb your appetite or hold you over until the next meal. More often than not, however, it is just a bad habit that can quickly devolve into binge eating. If you must have snacks, limit them to healthy foods in small portions.

Alcohol

Drinking alcohol lowers inhibitions and often ends in overeating. An alcohol fueled binge is particularly bad because there are a lot of calories in most forms alcoholic beverages. A night of drinking can mean consuming as many calories as a whole meal. Heavy drinking can cause you to take in more calories than you should in a full day worth of meals. Drinking less often and eating a good meal before drinking can help, but avoiding it as much as possible is best.

Giving up dieting is easy. Changing other bad habits is generally fairly easy also. A little planning ahead solves most of them the rest just need a good habit to replace them. The benefit from giving them all up is much improved ability to avoid bingeing episodes.

Dieting does not help. Many of us have been on diets our whole lives. We don't permanently lose weight on diets, and worse they keep us in a cycle of starving ourselves, then bingeing, then feeling ashamed and back to dieting. It is a trap that holds us back from doing the work that will actually heal us. Other bad habits have a similar effect. Eliminating bad food related habits clears the road of obstacles to better health. It is the start if building a plan for how you will eat going forward.

Chapter 4: **Create Sustainable Eating and Living Habits**

As we have seen, diets will not help you lose weight. They won't help you with binge eating either; in fact dieting can be part of the cycle that leads us into binge eating. When a diet fails us, we go into chaotic and unplanned eating. These are the times when we do the most damage to ourselves with food. Food choices are made in the moment and tend to be processed comfort foods. We crave the foods we were prohibited from eating in diet we just quit. Even if it doesn't taste good, we eat it in rebellion against the oppression of the diet. Chaotic eating isn't a solution, so what should we do? The answer is to be smart about how you eat. Choose good foods and plan meals in advance.

Diets fail because they are restrictive and take your favorite foods from you. Instead of taking foods away, add in high quality nutrient dense fresh foods. Eat enough of these foods to energize and satiate your body.

It is important to remember to find the healthy foods that you like to eat. Everyone likes the idea of kale, but nobody actually likes to eat kale. If you try to force yourself to eat it, you are tempting a backlash binge. Eating food should be pleasurable, not tedious. If you enjoy eating this way you will continue doing it. If not you won't. You are not limited to just healthy foods. Other less healthy foods can still be eaten, but they are no longer the focus of the meal. Since you can eat what you truly want, there is no restriction to rebel against. If you crave something you can have it, just make sure you take care of all your bodies nutritional needs first.

Planning your meals gives you ultimate control over your food intake. When you decide what you are going to eat ahead of time, you can choose foods that replenish and nourish you. You have more control over portion size when you pre plan a meal. Most people eat whatever is in front of them even if it is more than they really wanted. By setting a portion size before hand, you can reduce over eating. You can also control the amounts of processed foods you eat. This allows you to have the foods you crave but in smaller quantities mixed with nutritious foods.

Having a meal plan also includes deciding when to eat. As discussed previously, the timing of meals plays a role in avoiding triggers, as well as maximizing the use of the energy derived from the food. Spacing meals farther apart increases the number of calories burned, but also runs the risk of increased hunger and increased risk of binge eating. Finding a balance between the two is necessary and dependent on your goals. If weight loss is the primary reason for changing your eating habits, then spread out you meals more, especially the time between dinner and breakfast. If ending binge eating is your primary concern, shortening the time between meals would be better.

An important decision to make in your food plan is whether or not you want to allow snacking. Snacks can be trouble. When we binge eat, we don't consciously think about the food or eating it. In other words we are not mindful of our food. When you eat something you enjoy, the food should have your full attention. If you are mindlessly eating it and not even noticing it, why bother eating it at all? Snacking is usually not mindful eating. We eat something while we are working or watching television. This may be why snacking leads us into overeating so easily. But if you plan snacks, they are ok. Pre-portioned high quality and tasty snacks can hold you over between meals and keep you from getting to the ravenously hungry point where bingeing is inevitable. By having a food plan, you can make snacking a beneficial part of your daily routing. Without planning, snacking is an invitation to binge.

By planning the foods you eat and scheduling the times you eat them, you eliminate many of the pitfalls that lead to binge eating. You also give yourself the ability control your food intake and tailor it to accomplish the goals that you set. You decide if you want to tailor your plan to lose weight, manage overeating, or both.

Along with a food plan, a plan for getting enough sleep and exercise will make your eating plan much more successful. Sleep and exercise strengthen and replenish you.

Finding a form of exercise that you genuinely enjoy and scheduling yourself time to do it regularly further enhance your ability to control your eating and your life. Ideally you would do something that you like to do and look forward to. If it is something that you want to do, there is a much better chance of you continuing to do it.

Finally, getting enough sleep is necessary to get the full benefits from how you eat and exercise. A full night's sleep will allow you to lose weight. When you are sleep deprived, your body holds on to the weight, and it is extremely difficult to lose it. Exercise breaks down muscle and bone. The body repairs and strengthens muscle and bone best when you sleep. Good food, exercise, and proper sleep will help you look and feel your best. How you see yourself goes a long way toward how you treat yourself.

Now you have the tools to change how you eat and how you feel. You have control over many of triggers that spark binge eating. The effects of triggers not under your control can be muted or avoided entirely because of the plans you have in place. With these tools the drive to binge eat can be severely weakened or done away with entirely. The last part of the puzzle is maintaining the food plan and further insulating you from a possible relapse.

Chapter 5: **Self Acceptance and Avoiding Relapse**

Once you have your triggers under control and are eating healthy nourishing meals at regularly scheduled times and all is going well, how do you avoid a relapse? As discussed in earlier chapters, avoiding triggers is extremely important. But sometimes the triggers are difficult to avoid. Having a negative body image makes seeing yourself in the mirror a potential trigger. It's is pretty difficult to avoid yourself, so if negative body image is a trigger for you, then you'll have to find ways to improve how you see yourself.

Negative body image means feeling uncomfortable in your own skin. You don't believe you are attractive or are worthy of attraction from others. You feel anxiety and shame about the size of your body and you see yourself as a failure for allowing it to happen.

It can act as a trigger for some, but even if it doesn't directly lead to over eating and bingeing it can play a role in a relapse. When you feel good about how you look, doing the work to look and feel healthy is easier. If you don't like the way you look, it can drag down your mood and ability to make healthy choices. Maintaining a positive body image of ourselves is important to maintaining a binge free life. If, every time you see yourself in the mirror you get depressed, you may end up in an overeating cycle. This chapter is about improving body image and other ways to reduce the risk of backsliding into overeating.

The causes of negative body image are in large part due to the presentation of ideal bodies as normal in media. Children grow up in a world believing that the flawless bodies they see in media are what they should look like, and that they are flawed. We get caught up comparing ourselves to the perfect bodies we see, and we find ourselves lacking. Feeling this way about your body can make you feel overly self conscious in public. Negative feelings about your appearance are negative feelings about who you see yourself to be. There are ways to combat negative body image.

Accept Yourself for Who You Are

Nobody is perfect. You want to look like that actor or supermodel? It isn't possible. *They* don't even really look like that! Teams of trainers, dieticians, makeup artists, sleep therapists, plastic surgeons, and others are paid a lot of money to keep them looking as good as humanly possible. Even with all that help, and a professional photographer under perfect lighting, their pictures still get photo shopped. Perfection does not exist. These enhanced images of enhanced people are shown to you specifically to make you feel inferior, so that you will buy more products.

Ignore the Media

Avoid media offerings that only feature "ideal" body imagery and discussion. The advertising, fashion, and entertainment industries are not your friend when it comes to body image. Nothing will make you feel bad about your body image faster than comparing yourself to a six foot tall super model with amazing curves and a pencil thin waist, or that perfectly chiseled actor with the 6-pack. It's easy to fall into the trap. Images of perfect bodies are everywhere. But, if you look away from the magazine rack, television, or your phone and look at the people around you. They don't look like the people in those pictures either. They probably look a lot like you.

Focus on Positives

Find a couple of things about your body that you do like and focus on those things when negative thoughts come up. Better yet, try to see yourself through the eyes of someone who adores you. What is it they like about your body? Instead of berating yourself for imperfections focus on your positive qualities. Do the same for other people. There is no good reason to make negative comments about your body or other people's bodies either.

Get Some Exercise

Not only will exercise make you feel better and look better, it can make you feel strong and confident. Like with food choices, choosing a form of exercise you find enjoyable will make it easier to stick with it. Hiking, swimming, paddle boarding, team and individual sports, or anything else that will raise your heart rate and make you sweat a little bit. Ideally, you would find a challenging physical activity that you enjoy to the point that it becomes something you look forward to.

Exercise is very important to staving off binge eating even for those without body image issues. The strength and energy boost that comes with regular physical activity make it easier for you not need to overeat.

Get Some Sleep

Not getting adequate sleep can be damaging to body image. It can make you gain weight and it can make you look older and, well, tired. Sleep is rejuvenating. Your body repairs and restores itself while you sleep. You will look healthier because you'll be healthier. A full night's sleep can also invigorate the spirit as energy levels rise.

Cut Yourself Some Slack

Relapses happen. There is really no point in beating yourself up for falling off the wagon. Getting upset about a relapse puts you back into a shame cycle that got you here in the first place. Recognize that this is a difficult problem, and there will be setbacks, but that you are on a viable path to healthiness and you will succeed. All you can do is give yourself the best chance to succeed every day.

Take Care of Yourself

The way to beat binge eating is through self care. Caring for yourself with good food that satisfies all your body's needs and your need to enjoy what you eat. Getting enough sleep and exercise to make you healthier and happier is self care. Encouraging a positive body image is also caring for yourself by accepting and even liking who you are. So, take care of yourself and stay healthy!

Conclusion

Thank for making it through to the end of *Binge Eating: Guide to Stop and Overcome Overeating*, let's hope it was informative and able to provide you with all of the tools you need to achieve your goals whatever they may be.

The next step is to decide that you want to change your life. Are you ready to do the work necessary to make your life better? To get off the path that leads to obesity, diabetes, poor mental and physical health, and an early death? It starts with the will to change.

Now that you know why some foods and eating habits cause obesity and diabetes, you can make informed decisions on what to eat and how much. Factor in choosing what times you eat, and you have the ability to tailor you food plan to achieve the specific goals you have set. Whether you choose to lose weight, just steer clear of binge eating, or both, is up to you.

It sounds like a lot of work. Fortunately, the steps advocated in this book are relatively easy. You are not asked to give up foods you love or be expected to sweat in misery as you do exercises you hate. You are not asked to diet at all. Actually, you should quit dieting altogether. Dieting will not help you, and in fact it can hurt you, by causing you to rebel and go back to binge eating. Dieting is often part of the cycle of binge eating that is keeping you from living life to the fullest. For these reasons, dieting should be rejected.

Finding ways to heal yourself of bingeing that are sustainable- meaning they are enjoyable to do so it is easier to keep doing them, is the key to lasting life change and freeing yourself from overeating. You can change your life, and you now have the tools to do it.

So go out and live your best life. A life full of fun activity and healthy joyful eating that is worth living. Be free from binges and the shame and self harm that come with them. Enjoy being fully energized and healed by the food you eat, and not dragged down by it. Live in the confidence that you will succeed, even if you have a relapse, the path back to health is here for you. Be comfortable in your body and confident around other people without being victimized by negative body issues. Live as an example to others that binge eating can be conquered.

** Remember to use your link to claim your 3 FREE Cookbooks on Health, Fitness & Dieting Instantly

https://bit.ly/2Lvj2Pm

Printed in Great Britain
by Amazon